LICHEN SCLEROSUS DIET

Promoting Appropriate Dietary Health In Individuals With Lichen Sclerosus: Meal Prep & Planning

ERMIA GRIFFIN

Table of Contents

Introductory

Although it can appear everywhere on the body, the vaginal and anal regions are especially vulnerable to the chronic inflammatory skin disorder known as lichen sclerosus (LS). In this condition, the immune system mistakenly assaults healthy tissues in the body, hence the name "autoimmune disorder."

It is unclear what causes lichen sclerosus, although it is likely due to interactions between genes, hormones, and the immune system. It cannot be passed from person to person by casual touch, as it is not infectious.

Postmenopausal women, rather than men, are at increased risk for developing lichen sclerosus. But it can strike males of any age, females of any age, and even young toddlers.

White, flaky, thin, and brittle skin that is either wrinkled or glossy is the hallmark of this disorder. It has the potential to be itchy, uncomfortable, painful, and even scarring. Complications with urination, sexual activity, and other activities may arise if lichen sclerosus spreads to the vulva and causes the labia to narrow and fuse.

Although lichen sclerosus has no known medical solution, it can be treated to alleviate symptoms and prevent consequences. Topical corticosteroids, immune-modulating drugs, and moisturizing creams are all possible options for treating eczema. Consequences or related diseases, such skin cancer, can be caught early with regular medical screening.

Consult a medical expert for a proper diagnosis and treatment if you suspect you have lichen sclerosus or are experiencing symptoms.

CHAPTER ONE
Factors And Causes

It is unclear what exactly triggers lichen sclerosus (LS). However, there are a number of factors that may have a role in the onset of the illness. Among these are:

• Triggering factors: Lichen sclerosus is thought to be an autoimmune illness in which the immune system mistakenly targets healthy tissues. It is not yet known what sets off this autoimmune reaction.

• Hormonal considerations: In postmenopausal women, hormonal variables may contribute to the onset of LS. Decreased estrogen levels have been linked to skin that is both thinner and more prone to damage.

• Lichen sclerosus has been shown to have a hereditary component, as it often occurs in clusters within families. However, we still don't know the names of the genes responsible.

• Previous skin damage or trauma: Some experts believe that this may enhance the likelihood of developing lichen sclerosus in the damaged areas of skin. This may be the result of a past skin ailment, injury, or chronic irritation.

The possibility of acquiring lichen sclerosus can also be increased by other circumstances, in addition to those already mentioned:

• Although it is more frequent in postmenopausal women, lichen sclerosus can afflict people of any age or gender, including children. About ten times as many women as men are thought to be impacted.

• A higher chance of acquiring lichen sclerosus is associated with a family history of the disease.

• Lichen sclerosus is more likely to appear in people who have a history of other autoimmune illnesses, such as hypothyroidism or vitiligo.

• Long-term inflammation or infection: Genital or anal area infections that persist for an extended period of time may increase the risk of lichen sclerosus.

The presence of these risk factors does not ensure the onset of lichen sclerosus, but it does raise the possibility of it happening. Even if a person has all of the risk factors for LS, they may not end up developing the disease.

Diagnosis And Manifestations

Symptoms of lichen sclerosus (LS) vary from person to person and can be influenced by factors such as gender and age. Typical LS symptoms consist of:

• One of the most noticeable symptoms of lichen sclerosus is itching, medically known as pruritus. Scratching your itchy, uncomfortable skin can make it worse.

• Areas of skin that are white, shiny, and smooth often appear on people with LS. Atrophic, thinning, or wrinkled skin may form in certain areas. The skin may become delicate and prone to damage in these situations.

• Alterations to the skin: The affected area's skin may weaken and become more fragile over time. It may become wrinkled or reminiscent of cigarette paper. Scarring or discoloration of the skin may develop in more serious situations.

• Some people with LS may feel pain or soreness in the affected areas, especially when urinating or engaging in sexual activity.

• Women with LS may experience dyspareunia, or pain or discomfort during sexual activity.

• Urinary incontinence can occur if LS causes the labia to constrict or fuse, preventing normal urination.

• The afflicted skin may bleed or rip easily, especially during sexual activity or when scratched vigorously.

• Involvement of the anus: LS can also cause itching, soreness, or bleeding in the skin around the anus.

A dermatologist or other medical expert will often examine the damaged skin to make a diagnosis of lichen sclerosus. A biopsy is a small piece of skin tissue that is removed and examined under a microscope to confirm the diagnosis or rule out other possible causes.

If you have any of the signs of lichen sclerosus or think you might have the disease, you should see a doctor very away. Managing symptoms, avoiding complications, and increasing quality of life are all aided by prompt diagnosis and treatment.

CHAPTER TWO
Autoimmunity And Inflammation

The immune system's inflammatory response serves to defend the body from viruses, injuries, and irritants. Different types of immune cells, chemical mediators, and molecular signaling pathways all play a role in this intricate process.

Autoimmune illnesses, including lichen sclerosus, occur when the body's immune system assaults healthy tissues instead of harmful invaders. It causes persistent inflammation because the body's own cells and tissues are mistakenly identified as foreign or hazardous.

Tissue damage, functional impairment, and autoimmune disease symptoms can all come from inflammation.

The precise mechanisms that set off the autoimmune response and inflammation in lichen sclerosus are not well understood. However, it is thought that immune cells are called in, inflammatory mediators are released, and skin tissue is destroyed because the immune system recognizes certain components in the damaged skin as foreign.

Itching, white patches, and a general skin thinning are common signs of lichen sclerosus, which is caused by persistent inflammation. Scarring and structural alterations can develop in the affected areas when an inflammatory response has occurred for some time.

Treatments for autoimmune illnesses often seek to minimize inflammation and modify or suppress the immune response. Medication, including corticosteroids, immune-modulating medicines, and topical treatments, may be used to treat symptoms and delay the progression of the condition.

While inflammation is characteristic of autoimmune disorders, the specific causes and triggers can vary widely from one condition to the next. To better diagnose and treat autoimmune diseases like lichen sclerosus, researchers are working to identify the underlying causes and mechanisms that contribute to these conditions.

Causes And Effects Linked To Food Consumption

Some people who have lichen sclerosus (LS) say they notice an exacerbation of their symptoms when they consume particular foods or substances; nevertheless, the exact dietary triggers and aggravating factors for LS are not well-established.

It's worth noting, too, that LS symptoms and treatments can vary widely from person to person, and that there's scant scientific data to back up dietary advice. For specific advice, it's best to speak with a doctor or dermatologist. However, some persons with LS have observed that the following dietary factors worsen their condition:

• Meals high in oxalates, such spinach and rhubarb, can aggravate symptoms in certain people, as can spicy meals, acidic foods (like citrus fruits and tomatoes), and fatty foods. Keeping a food journal could be useful for pinpointing certain triggers.

• Inflammation can be triggered or made worse by food allergens or sensitivities in some people. Gluten, dairy, eggs, and soy are some of the most often encountered food allergies. An elimination diet or allergy testing can help you figure out which foods are causing or exacerbating your LS symptoms if you have reason to believe that they are doing so.

• While no definitive research has linked sugar or processed meals to LS, several sufferers have found that cutting less on these items has helped them feel better. The standard advice for optimal health is to eat a diet that is both healthful and balanced, with enough of whole foods.

• Coffee, tea, and other caffeinated drinks, as well as alcoholic beverages, may aggravate irritation and inflammation in certain people. Reducing or eliminating these substances to check for symptom improvement may be helpful.

• Varied foods and drugs may have varied effects on different people with LS due to individual differences known as triggers. Keeping track of how your body reacts to various foods and drugs can help you pinpoint any recurring patterns or triggers that might be exacerbating your symptoms.

It cannot be overstated how very individual the effect of nutrition is on LS symptoms; what helps one person may not help another. Consult a healthcare provider or dermatologist for individualized advice and guidance if you feel that certain foods or drugs may be exacerbating your LS symptoms. Together, you and your doctor can create a plan that is uniquely suited to your condition.

CHAPTER THREE
Nutritional Support For Lichen Sclerosus

Adopting a nutritious and balanced diet may have benefits for overall health and may help manage symptoms, but there is limited research addressing a diet that is lichen sclerosus (LS) friendly. The following are some guidelines that could prove useful:

• Eat lots of fruits and vegetables, whole grains, beans, and healthy fats like olive oil, nuts, and seeds to reduce inflammation in the body. Inflammation in the body tends to decrease after eating certain meals.

• Fatty fish (salmon, mackerel, sardines), flaxseeds, chia seeds, walnuts, and other foods rich in omega-3 fatty acids should be incorporated into your diet. Omega-3 fatty acids may aid in immune system regulation and have anti-inflammatory effects.

• Staying hydrated is important, so make sure to drink lots of water. Keeping yourself well hydrated is crucial to skin health and may help reduce the dryness and irritation caused by LS.

• Nutrient-dense foods are those that are high in many different nutrients, such as vitamins, minerals, and antioxidants. Colourful produce, lean meats, whole grains, and low-fat or non-dairy dairy products are all examples.

• Yogurt, kefir, sauerkraut, and kimchi are all great examples of probiotic-rich foods that you may want to include to your daily diet. Probiotics help maintain a balanced microbiota in the gut, which is important for proper immune system development and maintenance.

• Personalization is key because the causes and manifestations of LS in different people might vary widely. It may be possible to pinpoint specific food sensitivities or intolerances by keeping a food diary and making note of any possible trigger foods or symptom patterns.

However, dietary changes alone may not be enough to entirely relieve LS symptoms, and there is no universal solution. It is best to consult with a doctor or trained nutritionist who can tailor recommendations to your unique condition, health background, and set of personal triggers.

You should also stick to the treatment plan your doctor has laid out for you, which may involve topical treatments, immune-modulating pharmaceuticals, or other interventions designed to address your particular illness.

The Basics Of A Diet For Lichen Sclerosus

Although there is no medically-approved diet for lichen sclerosus (LS), eating well is an important part of leading a healthy life and may help with symptom management. Here are some general guidelines to follow when creating your LS diet:

• Include a wide selection of fruits and vegetables in your diet, especially those of different colours. They can aid in general wellness and immune system function because to their high vitamin, mineral, antioxidant, and fibre content.

• Select whole grains: Whole wheat, brown rice, quinoa, oats, and barley are some examples of whole grains that you should choose instead of refined grains. Blood sugar levels may be maintained with the help of whole grains due to their higher fibre and nutritional content and lower glycemic index.

• Add more lean protein to your diet by eating things like chicken, fish, beans, tofu, and low-fat cheese and milk. Repairing damaged tissues, building muscle, and maintaining a healthy immune system all require protein.

• Avocados, almonds, seeds, and olive oil are all examples of healthy fats that should be incorporated into your daily diet. These fats nourish the body and have anti-inflammatory properties.

• Consume a lot of water during the day to keep yourself from getting dehydrated. Adequate hydration helps maintain healthy skin and may reduce dryness and irritation from LS.

• Reduce your intake of processed meals and added sugars. Processed foods are typically heavy in unhealthy fats, salt, and added sugars. Too much sugar in the diet has been linked to inflammation and other health problems.

• Individualization is key because people experience LS differently and have different triggers. Keeping a food diary and noting how different meals effect your symptoms could be very instructive. As a result, you may be able to zero in on your own unique set of sensitivities and triggers.

The best way to determine if dietary changes are right for you is to speak with a healthcare provider or registered dietitian who can tailor recommendations to your unique requirements, medical history, and triggers. They can assist in formulating a strategy that takes into account both your general health and the management of LS.

CHAPTER FOUR
What To Restrict Or Not Eat

Although there is no agreed-upon list of foods to avoid or limit when dealing with lichen sclerosus (LS), some patients have found that consuming particular foods or substances can exacerbate their condition.

It's worth noting that people have different reactions to LS, and there isn't much research to back up any particular dietary recommendations.

But here are some broad suggestions that have helped some people with LS:

• Some people with LS report improvement in their condition after eliminating or greatly reducing their consumption of foods known to trigger allergic reactions or sensitivities.

Gluten, dairy, eggs, soy, and some nuts are among the most often encountered food allergies. An elimination diet or testing for food allergies can help you figure out what foods are causing or exacerbating your symptoms.

• Foods high in capsaicin or other inflammatory compounds (such as chili peppers) and foods high in acetic acid (such as citrus fruits, tomatoes, and vinegar) have been linked by some to an increase in itching and irritation in sensitive persons. If you notice that these foods are making your symptoms worse, keeping a food diary may help you determine whether or not they should be avoided.

• Although there is no definitive proof connecting LS and added sugars or processed foods, some people do find that limiting their consumption of these items helps reduce their symptoms. Inflammatory foods like these may be harmful to your health as a whole.

• Consuming caffeinated beverages (such coffee or tea) or alcoholic beverages may exacerbate itching or inflammation, according to some reports. If you find that avoiding or reducing these substances helps relieve your symptoms, that's good news.

• Personal triggers: Some people may react differently to foods or other drugs, and everyone's experience with LS is unique. Keeping a food diary and noting any patterns or triggers that tend to increase your symptoms can be very useful.

Keep in mind that these are only people's personal experiences being shared; what may work for one person may not work for another.

Consult a healthcare provider or trained dietitian for individualized advice and guidance if you feel that certain foods or substances may be exacerbating your LS symptoms. They will work with you to create a plan that is unique to your condition, health background, and personal triggers.

How To Make A Meal Plan And Stick To It

It can be good to organize meals around a balanced and nourishing diet that promotes general health and well-being when dealing with lichen sclerosus (LS). Some advice and suggestions are as follows:

• Eat a wide variety of fresh produce, whole grains, lean meats, and healthy fats, with a focus on complete, unprocessed foods. These aid in general health since they contain vital nutrients.

• Anti-inflammatory foods should be prioritized, thus things like fatty fish (salmon, mackerel, sardines), leafy greens, berries, nuts, and seeds should be incorporated into your diet. Consuming these meals has the potential to lessen inflammation.

• Meal preparation can be simplified by focusing on lean proteins, such as skinless poultry, fish, lentils, tofu, or low-fat dairy products. Protein is critical for immune system health and recovery.

• Select fiber-rich fare: increase your intake of whole grains, legumes, fresh fruits, and veggies. Fibre improves intestinal health, speeds digestion, and makes you feel full.

• Drink lots of water throughout the day to keep your skin hydrated and healthy. You can add some diversity to your diet by drinking herbal teas or infused water.

• Take into account potential individual triggers: Keep track of how your body reacts to various foods and make a note of any sensitivities or triggers that exacerbate your LS symptoms. You can tailor your diet to your needs by restricting or eliminating certain foods.

• Allot some time in advance for meal preparation and bulk cooking. This can make it easier to stick to your nutritional goals by ensuring that you always have healthful options available.

• Try new herbs, spices, and natural flavor enhancers to give your dishes more depth and diversity. This might add to the flavour and satisfaction of your meals.

• Consult a specialist: think about hiring a certified dietician who specializes in inflammatory illnesses and autoimmune diseases. They can provide you individualized advice, show you how to spot potential offender foods, and design a diet program just for you.

• While eating does have a role in general health, it is essential to keep in mind the importance of prioritizing self-care in all its forms. Managing stress, engaging in regular physical activity, and getting enough sleep all play a role in decreasing the severity of LS symptoms.

Keep in mind that LS can have varying effects on different people, so what works for one may not work for another. To effectively manage LS and improve overall health, it's crucial to tune into your body, pay attention to your symptoms, and collaborate with healthcare specialists.

CHAPTER FIVE
Recipes And Menu Examples

As a starting point for a diet that is friendly to lichen sclerosus, here are some sample meal plans and dishes that include nutritious, whole foods:

First Sample Menu:

• Egg whites, spinach, bell peppers, and tomatoes are incorporated into a veggie omelet and served for breakfast. Toast some whole grain bread and serve alongside.

• Greek yogurt with a handful of mixed berries and some chia seeds makes a healthy snack.

• For example, a typical lunch would consist of grilled chicken breast served with a salad of mixed greens, cucumber, and cherry tomatoes tossed in olive oil and lemon juice.

• Carrot sticks with hummus make a great snack.

• Herb-crusted fish baked in the oven with quinoa and steamed vegetables for dinner.

• Snack on some almonds or walnuts in the evening.

Second Sample Menu:

• Overnight oats with sliced bananas and honey drizzled on top, prepared with rolled oats, almond milk, and chia seeds.

• Almond butter on apple slices makes a healthy snack.

• Quinoa salad with roasted bell peppers, cucumbers, cherry tomatoes, and grilled chicken for lunch.

• Almond butter on celery sticks is a great healthy snack.

• For dinner, try skewers of grilled shrimp, zucchini, bell peppers, and brown rice.

• Before bed, have some herbal tea and a nibble of dark chocolate.

Some suggestions for meals that can be included in the plans are as follows:

1. Salad of mixed greens and grilled chicken:

• Sprinkle chicken breasts with seasonings such garlic powder, paprika, and thyme, or use your favourite blend.

• Cook the chicken completely on the grill.

• Put in a bowl some mixed greens, cucumber, cherry tomatoes, and other veggies of your choice.

• Use virgin olive oil, fresh lemon juice, salt, and pepper to dress the salad.

• Toss the grilled chicken with the salad and serve.

2. Quinoa and steamed broccoli accompanied by baked salmon.

• Set oven temperature to 400 degrees Fahrenheit (200 degrees Celsius).

• Salt, pepper, and any herbs you choose, such dill or lemon zest, should be used to season the salmon fillets.

• Bake the salmon for 12-15 minutes, or until it reaches an internal temperature of 145 F.

• Follow the package directions for cooking quinoa.

• Cook broccoli in a steamer until crisp-tender.

• Cook some quinoa and simmer some broccoli and serve it alongside the baked salmon.

Make sure to alter these menus and recipes to suit your tastes, food allergies, and other triggers. If you want specialized advice and to make sure the meal plan is going to satisfy your unique nutritional needs, it's best to go to a doctor or a qualified dietitian.

Sclerotized Lichen Need Certain Nutrients

Although there is currently no known treatment or cure for lichen sclerosus (LS), there is evidence to suggest that getting enough of a few key nutrients will help. Some of the most important nutrients to include in your diet are:

• Omega-3 fatty acids are anti-inflammatory and may aid in immune response modulation; they are found in fatty fish (salmon, mackerel, sardines), flaxseeds, chia seeds, and walnuts. Eating more of these foods may help reduce inflammation caused by LS.

• Vitamin D: Vitamin D has been shown to be important for immune function and to have potential anti-inflammatory effects.

Vitamin D can be obtained from a variety of food sources, including sunlight, fatty fish, fortified dairy products, and egg yolks, although sunlight is the best source. Your doctor may suggest taking vitamin D3 if you get very little sun and need to boost your vitamin D levels.

• Antioxidants are compounds that help shield cells from oxidative stress.

Antioxidants such as vitamins A, C, and E can be found in abundance in a diet that features a wide variety of fruits and vegetables. Good food sources include berries, leafy greens, citrus fruits, and vibrantly coloured veggies.

• Zinc: It helps with immunity and mending wounds. Zinc can be found in foods like seafood, beans, nuts, and seeds. Getting enough zinc in your diet may help your immune system and your body rebuild itself.

• Fibre: Getting enough fibre every day is important for digestive health and regular bowel motions. Increase your fibre intake by eating more fruits, vegetables, legumes, and whole grains.

• Vitamins B, like B6, B12, and folate, are essential to proper immune system function and nerve tissue maintenance. You can get B vitamins through meals like meat, fish, eggs, vegetables, beans, and fortified cereals.

• Probiotics are live microorganisms that help keep your digestive system and immune system healthy. Yogurt, kefir, sauerkraut, and kimchi are just a few examples of the many fermented foods that are rich in probiotics. Your doctor may also suggest taking a probiotic supplement.

You should still aim for a varied and balanced diet that caters to your specific needs, even if some nutrients may have some positive effects.

If you have dietary limitations, medical issues, or are thinking about taking supplements, it is essential that you speak with a healthcare practitioner or registered dietitian to receive individualized recommendations. They can personalize their advice to your specific needs and help you make sure you're getting enough of the nutrients your body requires.

CHAPTER SIX
Medicinal Herbs And Vitamins

Although there is scant research on the efficacy of herbs and supplements in treating lichen sclerosus (LS), some patients have experienced improvement after using these methods.

It is recommended that before beginning any new herbal treatments or supplements, you speak with a healthcare expert, as the effectiveness and safety of certain herbs and supplements may vary from person to person.

Herbs and supplements that are often recommended include:

• The gel extracted from aloe vera plants has potential anti-inflammatory and relaxing effects. It has anti-itch and anti-irritant properties and can be administered topically to the affected area. However, a patch test should be done first in case any users are allergic to or sensitive to aloe vera.

• Traditional uses for the flowering plant Calendula officinalis—more commonly known as marigold—include its anti-inflammatory and wound-healing effects. Topical application of calendula creams or ointments has been shown to reduce skin irritation.

• Melaleuca alternifolia, or tea tree oil, has been studied for its potential to kill bacteria and fungi. Some people with LS have claimed improvement after applying a mixture of tea tree oil and a carrier oil directly to their skin. However, a patch test should be done before using tea tree oil because it can irritate the skin.

• Vitamin E is an antioxidant that has been shown to aid in skin protection and healing. Vitamin E oil or lotions are helpful for some people when applied topically to sore spots.

Vitamin E oil that hasn't been tampered with should be used.

• Supplemental fish oil, which is rich in omega-3 fatty acids, may help people with LS because of its anti-inflammatory effects. Dietary sources of omega-3 fatty acids include fatty fish, flaxseeds, and chia seeds.

• Supplemental or dietary use of live cultures of beneficial bacteria, known as probiotics, has been shown to have positive effects on digestive tract and immune system health. Even though there isn't a lot of data on probiotics specifically for LS, they might help with your general health.

Keep in mind that these are only personal experiences, and the results may vary. Furthermore, some plants and supplements may have negative drug interactions or adverse effects.

Before adding any herbs or supplements to your LS management plan, especially if you have preexisting medical issues or are using drugs, you should always consult with a healthcare provider. They can tailor advice to your situation and help you make the most of the product.

Precautions And Recommended Dosages

Herbal and supplement therapy for lichen sclerosus (LS) should be carefully considered, with the priority always being on patient safety. Individual factors including age, overall health, and preexisting medical conditions or drugs used can affect the appropriate dosage and safety concerns for any given herb or supplement. Here are some broad rules of thumb to follow:

• Discuss your plans with a healthcare provider, a competent herbalist, or a naturopath before beginning any new herbal medicines or supplements.

They can tailor their recommendations to your unique needs by considering factors like your medical history and the medicines you're currently taking.

• Dosage should be taken exactly as instructed on the product label or by a qualified medical expert. Overdosing increases the risk of unwanted side effects and drug interactions.

• You can ensure the quality and purity of herbal medicines and supplements by purchasing them from renowned brands or sources. If you want to know that a product has been evaluated and certified for quality and safety independently, look for third-party testing and certifications like USP (United States Pharmacopeia) verification or NSF International certification.

• It is crucial to be aware of any individual sensitivities or reactions to particular plants or supplements. Check for adverse events and determine your particular response with a patch test or modest dose.

• Herbal supplements and pharmaceuticals used to treat LS and other disorders may interact dangerously in some cases. It's possible that some herbs can thin the blood, alter glucose levels, or counteract the effects of some prescription drugs.

Avoid negative drug interactions by telling your doctor about all the drugs, vitamins, and herbs you're currently taking.

• Keep an eye out for adverse reactions: Herbal and supplement use might cause some unwanted side effects, so it's important to keep an eye out for them. If you have any negative effects, you should stop using it and see a doctor.

• It is especially crucial to talk to a doctor before taking any herbs or supplements if you are pregnant or breastfeeding because of the potential dangers they could cause to your unborn child.

• Use for a long period of time: While some herbs and supplements are best used for a limited time, others can be used indefinitely.

However, there may be side effects or interactions with some supplements if used for an extended period of time. Consult your doctor regarding the recommended treatment length.

Keep in mind that everyone reacts differently to herbs and supplements, so what works for one person might not work for you. Safe and effective use need expert direction. If you want to use any herbal remedies or supplements, you should tell your doctor. This will help ensure that your care is well-coordinated.

CHAPTER SEVEN
Changing Your Way Of Life To Improve Your Health

Managing lichen sclerosus (LS) is just one example of how making some healthy lifestyle changes may have a profound effect on one's health and happiness. Some major alterations to one's way of life may contribute to better health:

• Keep your diet well-rounded by eating a wide range of fresh produce, cereals, proteins, and healthy fats. Eat less junk food, sweets, and salty snacks. Be sure to drink plenty of water throughout the day to maintain your body's fluid levels.

• Exercise or other forms of physical activity that suit your talents and preferences should be performed on a regular basis. To improve your heart health, muscle strength, and flexibility, you should do some form of cardiovascular exercise (like walking, running, or swimming) and some form of strength training (like weightlifting or resistance training). Before beginning an exercise regimen, it's important to talk to your doctor.

• Managing your stress is important since it can have a negative effect on your health in general and may make your LS symptoms worse. Deep breathing exercises, meditation, yoga, mindfulness, and relaxing hobbies and activities are all great ways to deal with stress. If you're feeling overwhelmed by stress or anxious, it may be time to talk to a mental health expert for help.

• Get the recommended amount of sleep each night, which is between 7 and 9 hours. Lack of sleep has been linked to impairments in immunity, mood, and general health. Make your bedroom conducive to sleep by dimming the lights, limiting screen time, and learning and using relaxation techniques.

• Quitting smoking is important for your health in many ways. Inflammation and circulation problems are only two of the many negative effects that smoking can have on health. To successfully quit smoking, you should get help from healthcare professionals, support groups, and smoking cessation programs.

• Consume alcohol in moderation; this means no more than one drink per day for ladies and no more than two drinks per day for males. Drinking too much alcohol is harmful to your health and can have lasting effects on your liver and immune system as well as your overall wellbeing. In moderation, and especially if it makes your LS symptoms worse, alcohol should be avoided.

• Try to stay within a healthy weight range by eating a nutritious, well-balanced diet and getting frequent exercise. The symptoms of LS may be affected by the inflammation and hormonal imbalances that might result from being overweight.

• Proper skin care includes avoiding harsh chemicals and allergens and only using mild, fragrance-free soaps on the affected region. Use a moisturizer on a regular basis to prevent dryness. Consult a doctor about the best skin care products to use in managing LS.

• Schedule checkups with your doctor on a consistent basis to keep tabs on your health, discuss your LS symptoms, and ask any questions you may have. Getting checked on a regular basis might help doctors spot any changes or difficulties with your health.

• Connecting with individuals who understand what it's like to live with LS can be a great source of emotional and informational support. Emotional support, coping methods, and useful information for managing the condition can all be gained through education and the sharing of experiences.

Changing your lifestyle should be tailored to your interests and needs. The best way to deal with LS and improve your health as a whole is to engage with medical experts including dermatologists, gynecologists, and other specialists.

Dealing With Causes Of Angry Outbursts

An important component of managing with lichen sclerosus (LS) is learning to recognize and avoid what sets off flare-ups. Here are some methods for recognizing triggers, controlling them, and reducing flare-ups:

• Maintain a diary to record your symptoms, daily activities, and any triggers for your condition. Take note of any shifts in your symptoms, such as itching, irritation, or inflammation. This can be useful in determining if any particular foods, activities, or items are contributing to the problem.

• Take steps to prevent or reduce exposure to probable triggers once they have been identified through your symptom diary. Soaps, detergents, textiles, tight clothing, perfumes, meals, and stress are just a few of the common allergens. The frequency and severity of flare-ups can be mitigated by limiting or eliminating exposure to triggers.

• Use moderate, fragrance-free soaps and stay away from harsh chemicals or allergens that might exacerbate LS symptoms instead. When washing the affected area, go for methods that are mild and won't irritate the skin.

Instead of rubbing something forcefully with a towel, pat it dry.

• Choose comfortable, breathable garments by opting for fabrics like cotton that allow air to circulate freely. Don't wear anything too snug or constricting, as this might lead to chafing and irritation.

• Keep the genital area clean and dry, since moisture there might exacerbate LS symptoms. Wash the area with mild soap or water and pat it dry gently. The genital area is not the place for powders, douches, or other harsh items.

• Maintaining a well-moisturized afflicted area will help alleviate dryness and itching, so do it often. Afterwards, apply an emollient or moisturizer that is hypoallergenic and fragrance-free. Applying moisture can calm the skin and lessen any irritation.

• Managing your stress is important because it may cause or worsen LS symptoms. Take deep breaths, meditate, do yoga, or do something relaxing whenever you feel your stress levels rising. Do something you enjoy, get regular exercise, and spend time with friends and family to relieve stress.

• While there is no one set diet for those with LS, you may find that avoiding certain foods helps. To determine which foods may be causing you discomfort, it may be helpful to keep a food diary.

You may decide to restrict or avoid particular foods if you find a link between them and flare-ups. For further information on this topic, it may be helpful to speak with a registered dietitian or other qualified healthcare practitioner.

• Maintain routine visits to your healthcare provider (e.g., a dermatologist or gynecologist) to keep tabs on your LS and talk about any worries or changes you've noticed in your symptoms. They can advise you on how to handle triggers and flare-ups, and modify your treatment plan if necessary.

Keep in mind that everyone has different LS-related triggers and reactions. You need to experiment to figure out what helps you the most. If your symptoms persist or worsen, it's best to see a doctor so they can help you find the best course of action.

CHAPTER EIGHT
Seeking Help From Experts

In order to effectively manage lichen sclerosus (LS) and provide complete care, it is crucial to seek professional support. These medical experts are here to lend a helping hand:

• A dermatologist is a medical doctor who focuses on skin care and may provide expert diagnosis and treatment for LS and other skin conditions. They will be able to diagnose your disease correctly, recommend appropriate treatments, and keep tabs on your recovery.

• Because genital areas are so frequently affected by LS, a

gynecologist is an important medical specialist to see. They are able to give specialized care for genital LS, including regular inspections and treatment recommendations.

• If your LS has affected your urinary system or if you are experiencing urinary symptoms, it may be helpful to see a urologist. Any urinary issues caused by LS can be evaluated and treated.

• Your primary care doctor (PCP) is crucial in coordinating your healthcare as a whole. They can aid in the diagnosis of LS, make early treatment suggestions, and recommend further specialized care if required. They are able to provide care for the whole person, not just their specific ailment.

• When LS affects the pelvic region, a pelvic floor physical therapist can give specific therapy to alleviate pelvic pain and discomfort. They can aid with pain management, strengthening of the pelvic floor muscles, and better overall coordination.

• Although there is no established LS diet, a certified dietitian can offer advice on how to eat healthily and sustainably in general. They are useful for addressing targeted dietary issues like pinpointing allergenic foods and improving nutrient absorption.

It's important to be honest with your doctors about your LS symptoms, worries, and desired course of therapy. They are able to offer individualized guidance, several courses of treatment, and continuous care. Seek out doctors that have experience with or knowledge of treating LS or related disorders if at all possible.

In addition to medical help, people living with LS can benefit from interacting with others in similar situations through support groups or online communities. Talking to people who get you can be a great source of strength and solace.

Never disregard the counsel of a qualified medical expert who can assess your unique circumstances and provide tailored recommendations. With their assistance, you can get a treatment plan that works for you and learn to live with LS.

Holistic Treatments That Go Beyond Diet

Some people with lichen sclerosus (LS) find relief from a variety of complementary therapies and changes to their way of life. These methods should not replace standard medical treatment and should only be used after consulting with a doctor. Some holistic strategies to think about are as follows.

• Meditation, deep breathing exercises, yoga, tai chi, and mindfulness are just a few examples of mind-body practices that can aid in these areas and more. By lowering inflammation and boosting immunological function, these methods may aid with LS symptom management.

• Acupuncture is a traditional Chinese medicine practice that includes inserting very tiny needles into the body at strategic spots. Acupuncture has been reported to help alleviate the pain and itching experienced by some people with LS. Seek the advice of a licensed acupuncturist who has experience managing LS and similar symptoms.

• Herbal medicine: There is some evidence that certain herbal medicines, such as those with anti-inflammatory or immune-modulating qualities, can help those with LS.

However, if you want to make sure you're using herbal medications correctly and safely, it's best to talk to a professional herbalist or naturopath. They will be able to tailor their care to your individual needs and take into account any drug interactions.

• Reducing your stress levels can help your LS symptoms. Take advantage of stress-reduction strategies like regular exercise, hobbies, time in nature, and professional therapy. Discover what helps you feel more relaxed and optimistic.

• Some people with LS report improvement after applying a certain essential oil topically. Essential oils such as lavender, tea tree, chamomile, and calendula are frequently suggested as having possible anti-inflammatory and calming effects. Essential oils have many benefits, but it's important to use them with caution, dilute them, and do a skin test to be sure you're not allergic.

• Physiotherapy for pelvic floor dysfunction and pain is a viable treatment option for some people with LS. Physical therapy for the pelvic floor can help with a variety of conditions, including strengthening and improving coordination of muscles and relieving pain or discomfort caused by LS.

• Art therapy, journaling, and support groups are all examples of supportive therapies that can help individuals feel more connected to others and less alone in their struggles. These treatments can be helpful in managing the symptoms of a chronic illness like LS.

Keep in mind that holistic treatments are meant to work in tandem with standard medical care, not in place of it. Make sure these methods are acceptable for your unique circumstance and won't conflict with any current therapies by having a conversation with your healthcare providers.

Because everyone's time with LS is different, the strategies that work for some may not be appropriate for others. It's vital to tune in to your body, try out new methods, and get advice from medical experts who can tailor their suggestions to your specific situation.

Conclusion

The chronic nature of lichen sclerosus (LS) necessitates in-depth medical attention. Although there is currently no cure for LS, many people have found that medication, changes in lifestyle, and holistic practices have helped them manage their symptoms, speed their recovery, and improve their overall health.

Developing a personalized treatment strategy requires close collaboration with medical experts like dermatologists, gynecologists, and others.

Dietary changes, such as adhering to a diet designed for those with lichen sclerosus, may help with symptom management. Foods that may act as triggers should be avoided or limited, while anti-inflammatory and nutrient-rich foods should be incorporated, and a healthy lifestyle should be maintained.

Improvements to one's health can be achieved through a combination of dietary and other lifestyle changes. Taking care of LS requires a multifaceted approach that includes regular exercise, stress management, plenty of restful sleep, and diligent attention to personal hygiene.

To effectively manage LS, seeking professional guidance is crucial. Accurate diagnosis, treatment choices, and continuing monitoring of LS can be provided by dermatologists, gynecologists, urologists, primary care physicians, and other healthcare experts.

Counselors, nutritionists, and physiotherapists who specialize in treating the pelvic floor can all be helpful in coping with the mental and physical challenges of living with LS.

It is recommended to discuss the use of mind-body practices, acupuncture, herbal medicine, and supportive therapies with a medical practitioner to guarantee their safety and efficacy.

It's important to keep in mind that the symptoms and severity of LS vary from person to person, and that it may take some trial and error to determine the best course of action for managing your symptoms.

It is possible to improve LS management, increase well-being, and lead a full life by using a holistic approach, collaborating closely with healthcare experts, and making educated decisions.

THE END

19131904R00056